T0245275

Non Invasive
Mechanical Ventilation

Junaid Malik, MD, D. ABSM

Copyright © 2018 by Junaid Malik, MD, D. ABSM. 786610

ISBN: Softcover   978-1-9845-6878-6
         Hardcover   978-1-9845-6879-3
         EBook   978-1-9845-6877-9

Library of Congress Control Number: 2018914079

All rights reserved. No part of this book may be reproduced
or transmitted in any form or by any means, electronic
or mechanical, including photocopying, recording, or by
any information storage and retrieval system, without
permission in writing from the copyright owner.

Print information available on the last page

Rev. date: 12/03/2018

To order additional copies of this book, contact:
Xlibris
1-888-795-4274
www.Xlibris.com
Orders@Xlibris.com

TABLE OF CONTENTS

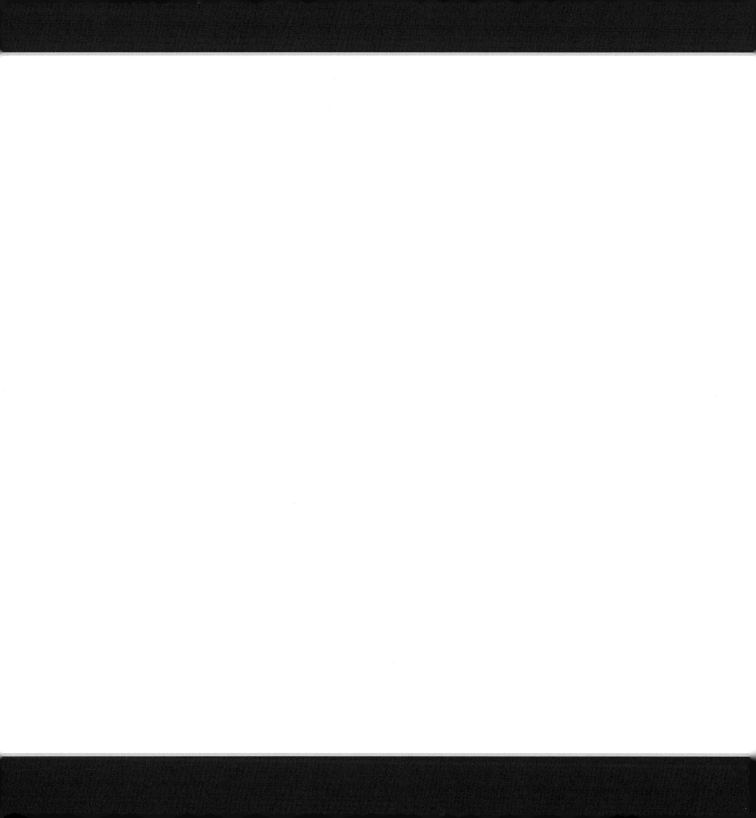

CHAPTER 1

I find it very interesting over years of practice to find sleep physicians or pulmonologists who prescribe positive airway pressure (PAP) therapy and not be able to actually change or look at the machines that they give to their patients. As technology advances, the provider has delineated this task to a durable medical equipment (DME) company, who tends to have a respiratory therapist or (at least) a driver to set up the patient with these PAP therapies. This is equivalent to going to a computer store to buy a computer and the sales representative does not even know how to turn on the computer you are about to purchase.

Technology advances, and learning these PAP or noninvasive mechanical ventilation (NIMV) devices is becoming more demanding; however, as a physician, this is as important as learning the next new electronic medical system. It is not very hard, and there are only about three to four main device companies.

One of the difficulties of using these machines is the lack of standardization of the nomenclature of various settings—for example, the interchangeable use of IPAP and pressure, which leads to difficulty in communicating between the physician and the DME company. At times this can be challenging and can potentially lead to erroneous settings of these devices. I have seen this issue arise when giving settings order for iVAPs and the DME is setting up an AVAPS. This worrisome problem extends to the fact that the DME company, which is usually determined by insurance, will use a certain device manufacturer and not even know about the other. Also, there is usually a high turnover rate in DME companies, which means that the respiratory therapist who sets up machines is different from the one a month ago and may not be as experienced.

This problem is not limited to DME companies only; it has been observed even in the inpatient settings. As onboarding of new equipment and devices occurs in many hospitals, the purchasing department may not inform the respiratory department about the incoming devices. This may lead to respiratory departments not even knowing the full extent of the devices' capabilities. They may have a respiratory therapist who uses an AVAPS machine only as a bilevel and does not understand the potential of such a machine. Also, the physician may not have any input and may also lack the full understanding of the machine being used in the hospital. I have learned over the years that my patients with NIMV may be hospitalized in another hospital but will not be allowed to use their NIMV in that facility as their respiratory department has no comprehension of the device.

In this manuscript, I am hoping to allow physicians and respiratory therapists to have a reference guide and possibly some understanding of the various NIMV units that are commonly available.

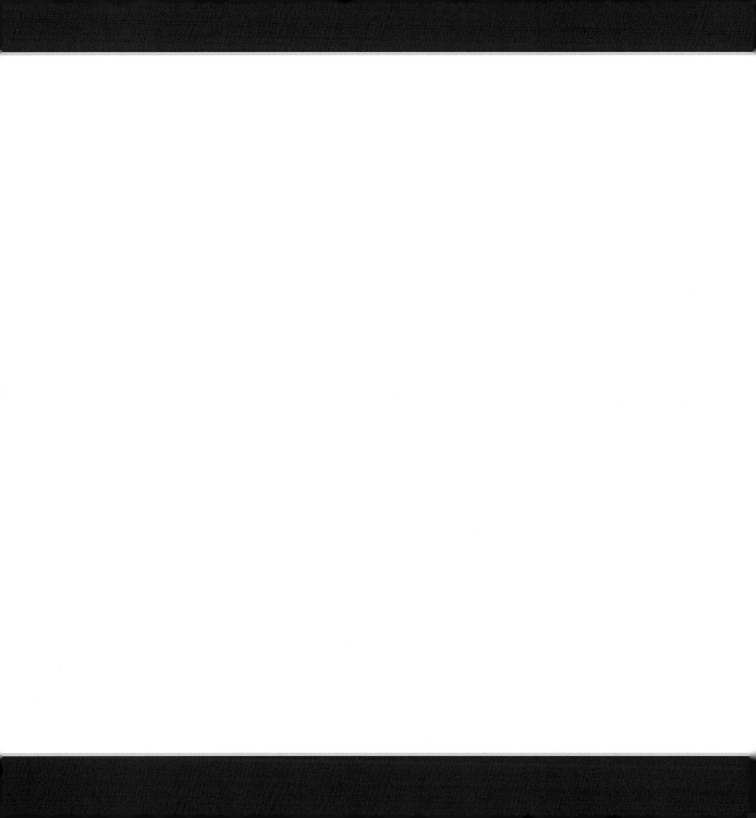

CHAPTER 2
The Mask

I think the most important and crucial part of NIMV is the interface between the machine and the person. Studies have shown that mask selection allows patients to benefit from and tolerate the pressures and interaction of the NIMV. There are about five basic mask types: (1) nasal pillow, (2) nasal mask, (3) NasOral mask, (4) full face mask, and (5) entire-head or helmet mask.

Cochrane's review on CPAP delivery interfaces for OSA concluded that nasal pillows may be a useful alternative to nasal masks and that full face masks could not be recommended as first-line choices.[10] However, there are limited number of studies to compare these mask types.

Most of the articles related to the fitting of masks for CPAP therapy, however, said that much can be derived from these studies and the potential application to NIMV. Rafaela and colleagues found that "most studies showed that oronasal masks are less effective and are more often associated with lower adherence and higher CPAP abandonment than are nasal masks."[1] In this same study, the concept of why a nasal mask may be more effective than oronasal mask, which may cause more obstruction, is shown in the following diagram.

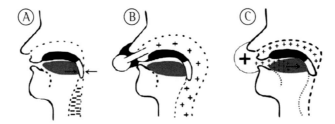

Figure 3 – In A, schematic illustration of the normal upper airway (left) of a patient with obstructive sleep apnea, showing retropalatal obstruction during negative pressure generated during inhalation (center) and during continuous positive airway pressure (right). In B, schematic illustration of a patient wearing an oronasal mask, and, in C, patient with significant mouth breathing. The tongue (red) is displaced posteriorly and obstructs the upper airway. Adapted from Sullivan et al.[21] Source: Schorr et al.[31]

Ebben et al.[5] found that switching from a nasal mask to an oronasal mask after titration resulted in increased residual AHI and may warrant a pressure adjustment. Bettinzoli et al. found that oronasal masks left more residual events than nasal masks and led them to conclude with the recommendation that nasal masks must be used first line in the treatment of OSA. A more recent study by Deshpande et al.[3] showed in patients with OSA that oronasal masks were associated with higher CPAP pressures compared to nasal mask types.

Patients and physicians believe that people are meant to keep their mouths open at night; thus, we need to have a full face mask. However, we are born as obligated nose breathers in order to be able to suckle as neonates and infants. Infants are obligate nasal breathers until at least two months old.[13] As humans mature, we learn to breathe through the mouth as we get nasal obstructions and other sinus issues. This fallacy about full mask has not been studied extensively, however Cochran review concluded "the nose mask performed better than the face mask (which covers both the nose and mouth) with one study showing greater compliance and less sleepiness, and was the preferred mask in almost all patients."[14]

The Masks

Nasal pillows: ResMed

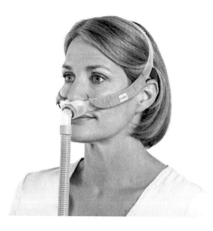

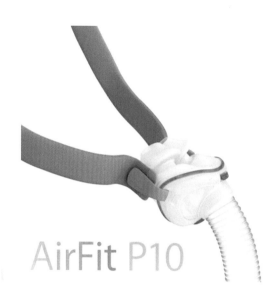

Respironics nasal pillows

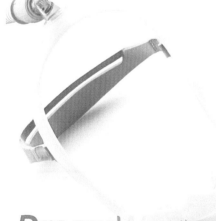

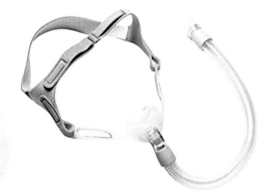

Fisher & Paykel nasal pillows

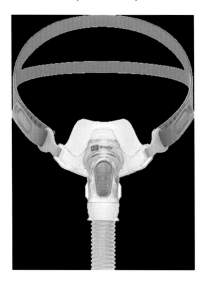

Nasal masks

Respironics

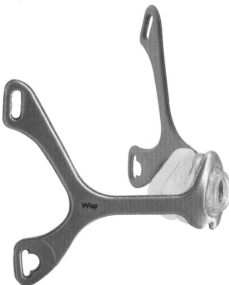

ResMed

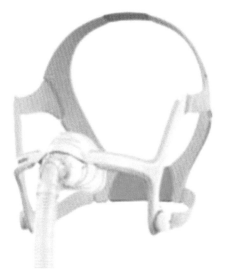

Fisher & Paykel nasal mask

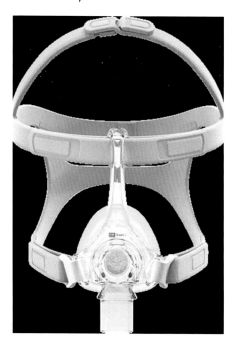

Respironics full face mask

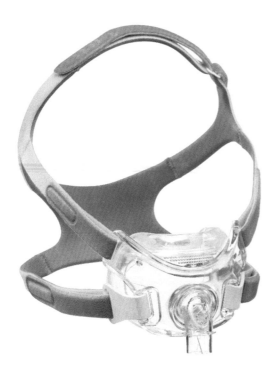

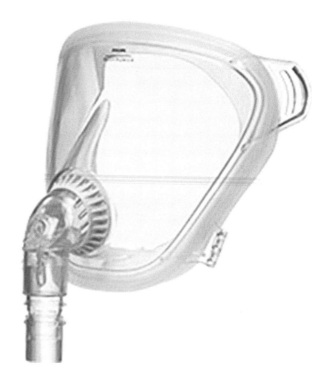

ResMed

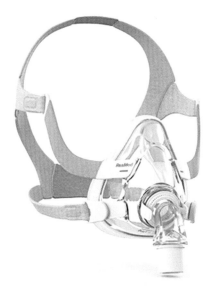

Fisher & Paykel oral-only mask

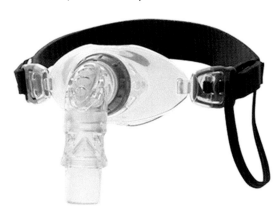

Fisher & Paykel

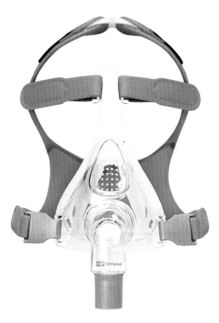

CHAPTER 3
Where Can You Use the NIMV?

As hospitals and physicians are graded on complications and readmissions of patients with more complex diseases, we are forced to integrate technology into the practice of medicine. We have already moved from the written medical record to the electronic medical record in the hopes of bettering the streamline of data and the interaction between physicians and the continuation of medical records. The realm of COPD has seen the changing of the GOLD guidelines and medications—however very little—on incorporating positive airway therapy.

Salturk et al.[6] has shown that after one year of using NPPV / NIMV (noninvasive mechanical ventilation) in patients with chronic or hypercapnic respiratory failure, there was a significant improvement in exercise capacity as measured by the six-minute walking distance.

Recently, Patrick MP et al.[11] showed to patients who were discharged home after acute exacerbation of COPD that adding home noninvasive ventilation to home oxygen therapy prolonged the time of readmission or death within twelve months. As the mounting evidence for use and understanding of NIMV becomes more practical and expanded, we, as clinicians, must understand and learn to use these new devices.

CHAPTER 4
The Machines: CPAP or Bilevel

ResMed
ResMed was founded in Australia and is now based in San Diego, California, USA.

Respironics
Phillips Respironics is based in Murrysville, Pennsylvania, USA.
Fisher & Paykel is based in New Zealand.

CPAP and AutoPAP

Continuous positive airway pressure (CPAP) is the most commonly used positive airway pressure (PAP) therapy. We know that CPAP is set with a pressure of 5–20 cm of water pressure (CWP). The AutoPAP, on the other hand, is given a range of 5–20 CWP; and then the machines will determine the appropriate pressure based on the resistance in the airway.

Some of the comfort features available in CPAP therapy are ramp, EPR, and A-Flex/C-Flex. The ramp allows the pressure to start at a lower pressure and, over a set time, increases the pressure to the set pressure in CPAP mode and the pressure range in the AutoPAP mode. There is also a feature called EPR (ResMed: expiratory pressure release) or A-Flex/C-Flex (Respironics: A for "auto" and C for "constant"). This allows the machine to release the CPAP pressure during exhalation. This range is between 1 and 3. It has the greatest benefit with higher CPAP settings.

Some of the areas of advancement now occurring are in the way we can monitor machines and access information about the various devices. ResMed has an Airview.Resmed.com website, which can access all the newer AirSense 10 device platforms. Respironics has an EncoreAnywhere.com website that will be upgrading to the CareOrchestrator.com website, which is available on the DreamStation platform. This will add a more streamlined approach to patient care and to interaction with the physician. For example, the patient may contact the physician and say that he/she needs an increased or decreased pressure on his/her CPAP/bilevel devices, and the physician can access the respective website and change pressures without having to place an order to the DME and assume that the order has been completed. These types of changes can be made in a few seconds as long as the physician is willing to adapt to the new access.

BiPAP and Auto BiPAP or Bilevel Therapy

BiPAP is trademarked (serial number is 7515449 and registration number is 2071585 in RIC Investments LLC); therefore, *bilevel* is a more appropriate word to use as to not cause issues with trademark.

Bilevel therapy is set as inspiratory (IPAP—inspiratory positive airway pressure) and expiratory (EPAP—expiratory positive airway pressure) pressure. This allows patients to breathe in a more normal pattern of breathing. The difference is usually set by the physician based on an unverified pressure difference, usually in a 3–5 CWP range, rather than asking the patient a simple question: "How deep of a breath do you want?" Most patients are able to answer this question. Once this is set, then a patient may have this adjusted to allow for appropriate ventilation.

The auto bilevel is given at an IPAP maximum and EPAP minimum and then in the ResMed pressure support at a difference between 1 and 10 CWP, and the Respironics pressure is usually set as minimum and maximum 1–8 CWP. This allows these auto bilevel devices to ventilate the patient based on the resistance in the airway. The algorithm that the Respironics auto bilevel uses to determine the adequate difference between the IPAP and EPAP is not completely understood by the author. However, the ResMed unit is set differently. These machines will usually give a compilation of data into a relatively easy document to assess the 90%–95% pressures, tidal volume, AHI, and leak. Therefore, a practitioner could adjust the IPAP maximum and EPAP minimum and pressure support into a more steady or narrower working pressure.

Comfort measures in the ResMed are ramp time and inspiratory time with a minimum of 0.1 to a maximum of 3.0 sec. The other comfort parameters are trigger and cycle. The trigger, which allows the machine to adjust its response to the initiation of inspiration, is set from very low to very high. The cycle is the response of the machine to expiration, and sensitivity is set from very low to very high. The trigger and cycle may need adjustments to keep the machine able to sense inspiration and expiration and allow easy breathing.

The trigger and cycle can be explained by the following diagrams from ResMed's website.[8] The trigger is the top diagram, and the cycle is the bottom diagram.

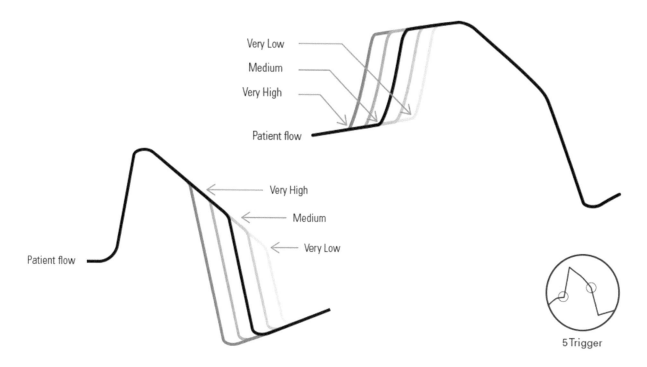

Comfort measures in the Respironics are ramp time, rise time, and inspiratory time. Ramp time and inspiratory time are the same as the ResMed machine. The rise time is the slope of inspiration, and this can be adjusted to allow for breathing. The rise time is the time between the start of inspiration and achievement of IPAP pressure. Using shorter inspiratory rise times will decrease the inspiratory workload.[7]

The AASM has given guidelines[2] for the sleep center titration of NPPV; however, these recommendations are for bilevel with backup rates.

These guidelines[2] provide an algorithm.

Figure 3—Schematic of NPPV titration protocol

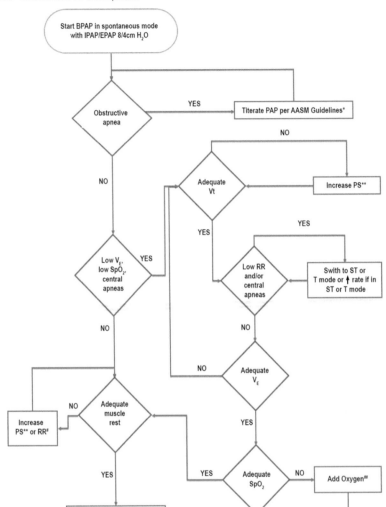

RR refers to respiratory rate; Vt, tidal volume; V_E, minute ventilation; SpO_2, oxyhemoglobin saturation by pulse oximetry; PAP, positive airway pressure; PS, pressure difference between EPAP and IPAP; ST, spontaneous timed mode; T, timed mode. *refer to section 1.4 and reference 48; **Increase PS 1-2 cm H_2O every 5 minutes (section 4.4); #Add NPPV initiated breaths at 1-2 breaths per minute below the NPPV naïve rate or increase RR 1-2 every 10 minutes (section 4.5); ##Add oxygen at 1 L/min or increase by 1 L/min every 5 minutes (section 4.7).

These guidelines[2] do have a section that includes volume-targeted bilevels with an initial target of tidal volume settings of 8 ml/kg ideal body weight. The purpose of sleep center titration in these machines is to adjust for EPAP settings and to allow the machine to adjust the IPAP maximum and minimum for tidal volumes.

CHAPTER 5
Advanced Assured Ventilation

The more advanced settings are iVAPS and AVAPS and AVAPS-AE. These modes of ventilation incorporate more settings and variables to adjust and to allow for comfort. These modes are in machines that are based on these modes and also in more advanced machines (i.e., Astral and Trilogy, respectively).

These advanced modes of ventilation—iVAPS and AVAPS—are targeting a certain alveolar ventilation or tidal volume, respectively, and adjusting pressure (i.e., pressure support or IPAP minimum and maximum) to achieve this volume. These machines will adjust the pressure from breath to breath or over a series of breaths. If the patients are apneic, the machine will institute a breath to achieve the set rate. However, these modes are more of an augmentation.

The Astral by ResMed

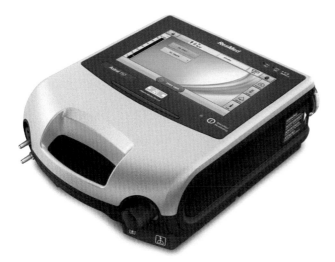

Accessing the menu: first, the menu will start by depressing the lock button located in the upper left corner of the screen. Then the next screen will appear.

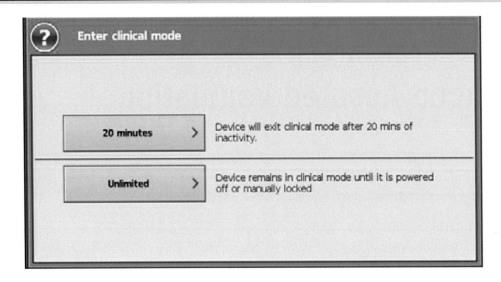

At this screen, pick either 20 min or unlimited time. I usually use unlimited so I will not have to keep unlocking the menu.

Once the Astral is unlocked, the next screen will appear.

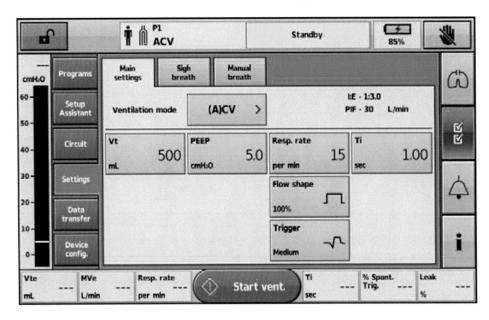

On the right of the menu is the following: , which is the monitoring button; then , which is the settings button; then , which is the alarm button; and finally, , which is the information button. The allows one to access the menu button for programs, setup assistant, circuit, settings, data transfer, and device configuration. These are located on the left-hand side of the setup menu. In the above setting, the settings button on the right has been pressed and the settings button on the left has also been pressed, allowing one to change the mode of ventilation. To change the mode of ventilation, depress the button that is shown above as (A)CV >. Then scroll through the settings until you find the setting that is right for your patient. We will be using the iVAPS > mode.

The iVAPS mode is made by ResMed. This mode is based on pressure regulation to achieve an alveolar ventilation. The EPAP is set to achieve the opening pressure of the throat. The EPAP should be thought of as CPAP; this allows us to break these machines down into small areas of influence.

Next is the alveolar tidal volume (TVa). This is the alveolar ventilation we want to achieve with each breath based on the height of the patient. Since alveolar ventilation can be measured directly, ResMed employs an algorithm based on estimation of anatomical dead space.[9]

This is the goal tidal volume that the machine will try to achieve.

When using the Astral platform, I have assumed that it will be used in the single-limb circuit with intentional leak.

The PS, or pressure support, is used with minimum and maximum. This is used by the machine to achieve the TVa. Initially, the pressure support minimum could be set at 2 CWP, and the maximum could be set at 15–20 CWP. This may need to be adjusted for the comfort of the patient. The basis of adjustment should be determined or considered with the 95% pressure for inspiration or PIP. Through clinical experience, this is where one should adjust the minimum PS set to where the PS is at 95% of time. In the following example, the EPAP is set at 5 and the minimum PS was initially set at 2; however, the PIP (positive inspiratory pressure) was seen at 9. I had to reset the minimum PS to 4 to make the IPAP be 9 CWP.

The other data obtained from this report: The patient has been 100% compliant with use of 10 h a day. The patient is using a nasal mask. AHI is 0.3, leak is at 8.9 L/min (liters per minute), and the tidal volume is 364 mL. The patient is comfortable and is using it without issues. Most importantly, the patient is not being hospitalized for acute episodes of respiratory failure.

The patient's PS may need further adjustment for the patient's comfort. Also, the TVa may need further adjustment based on the patient's comfort. These adjustments may need to be changed on a regular basis.

Compliance Report: Program 1

Usage: Program 1	11/23/2017 - 12/22/2017
Usage days	**30/30 days (100%)**
>= 4 hours	30 days (100%)
< 4 hours	0 days (0%)
Usage hours	326 hours 46 minutes
Average usage (total days)	10 hours 54 minutes
Average usage (days used)	10 hours 54 minutes
Median usage (days used)	11 hours 8 minutes

Astral 100: Program 1	SN: 22171117710
Device Settings: Program 1	
Mode	iVAPS
Circuit	Single with leak
Patient Interface	Mask
Mask	Nasal
Patient Type	Adult
Height	59.1 in
Inspiratory Phase Delivery Settings: Program 1	
Target alveolar ventilation	3.2 L/min
Min PS	4 cmH2O
Max PS	20 cmH2O
Rise time	500 ms
Inspiratory Trigger Settings: Program 1	
Target patient rate	18 breaths/min
Trigger	Medium
Inspiratory Phase Duration Settings: Program 1	
Ti Min	0.5 sec
Ti Max	1.5 sec
Cycle	40.0 %
Expiratory Phase Settings: Program 1	
EPAP	5 cmH2O

Therapy: Program 1					
Leak - L/min	5th %:	2.4	Median:	8.9	95th %: 23.7
Events per hour	AHI:	0.3	AI:	0.0	HI: 0.3

AirView™

Therapy Report: Program 1

Age: 78 years

Astral 100   SN: 22171117710

Usage: Program 1 (hours)

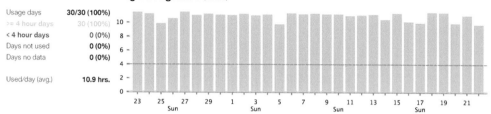

Usage days	**30/30 (100%)**
>= 4 hour days	30 (100%)
< 4 hour days	**0 (0%)**
Days not used	**0 (0%)**
Days no data	**0 (0%)**
Used/day (avg.)	**10.9 hrs.**

Leak: Program 1 (L/min)

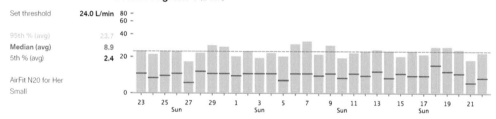

Set threshold	**24.0 L/min**
95th % (avg)	23.7
Median (avg)	8.9
5th % (avg)	2.4
AirFit N20 for Her Small	

Pressure: Program 1 (cmH2O)

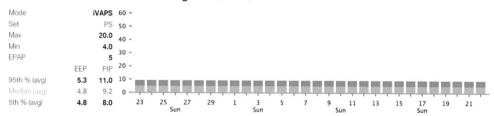

Mode			**iVAPS**
Set			PS
Max			**20.0**
Min			**4.0**
EPAP			**5**
		EEP	PIP
95th % (avg)		**5.3**	**11.0**
Median (avg)		4.8	9.2
5th % (avg)		**4.8**	**8.0**

AHI: Program 1 (events/hour)

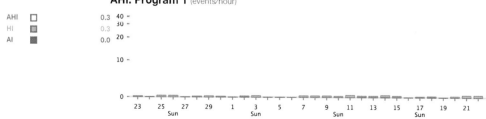

AHI	☐	0.3
HI	▣	0.3
AI	■	0.0

AirView™

Therapy Report: Program 1

Age: 70 years

Astral 100	SN: 22171117710

Tidal Volume: Program 1 (ml)

95th % (avg)	574
Median (avg)	364
5th % (avg)	119

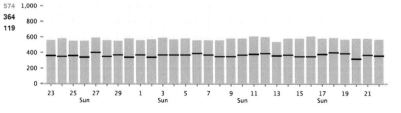

Respiratory Rate: Program 1 (breaths/min)

Target patient rate	18
95th % (avg)	24
Median (avg)	15
5th % (avg)	13

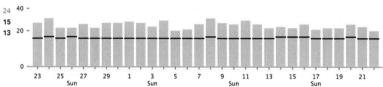

Minute Ventilation: Program 1 (L/min)

95th % (avg)	8.6
Median (avg)	5.6
5th % (avg)	4.2
Alveolar Ventilation	
95th % (avg)	7.3
Median (avg)	4.6
5th % (avg)	3.4

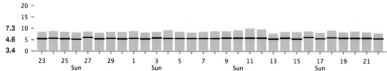

I:E Ratio: Program 1 (median in %)

95th % (avg)	2.97:1
Median (avg)	1:2.50
5th % (avg)	1:10.00
E%	
I%	

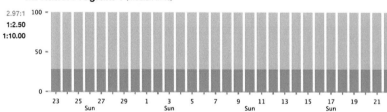

The next factors to be considered are the trigger and the cycle. Like the other bilevel devices, the trigger is set at low, medium, high, and very high. ResMed[9] provides a graphic representation that can help with better understanding the trigger function. My general rule is, most individuals without neurological issues will want a medium to very low sensitivity. However, those with neurological limitations may need to have the sensitivity set at high or very high in order for the machine to start the initiation of breath. This may need further adjustment with any neurological disorder as the disease process progresses.

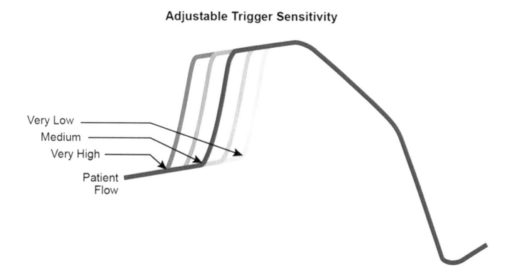

Once the trigger has been adjusted, then the cycle may need further adjustment. The cycle, on the other hand, is based on how quick or sensitive the machine needs to be in order to start the exhale of the patient. In general, the higher the sensitivity percentage, the quicker the machine will initiate the exhale. Again, the above rule that I use for the trigger is used with cycle sensitivity. The following flow diagram[9] should give a better insight into this setting. There is one constraint on the cycle: the Ti Min and Max. The inspiratory period cannot be less than Ti Min or longer than Ti Max.[9]

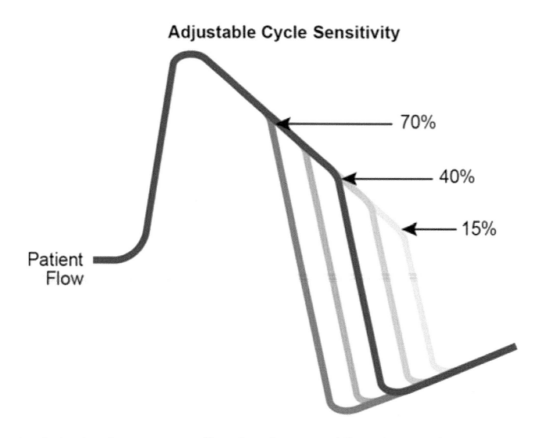

Adjustable Cycle Sensitivity

The rise time is the time from initiation of breath to the maximal flow. This is set from minimum to 500 ms (milliseconds). A general rule of thumb is to adjust this during the initial process of NIMV. A more anxious patient prefers a faster rise time of minimum or 150 ms. If you need more time to inspire, then I recommend increasing the Ti Max and also increasing the rise time to 300–400 ms; however, this adjustment is very patient dependent.

The flow-shape settings can easily be addressed. This setting can be used at times but is more commonly used with invasive mechanical ventilation. The following diagrams from the Astral guide better explain the settings.[9]

Flow shape settings

The Astral device supports four flow shape settings:

1. 100% (Constant)
2. 75%
3. 50%
4. 25%

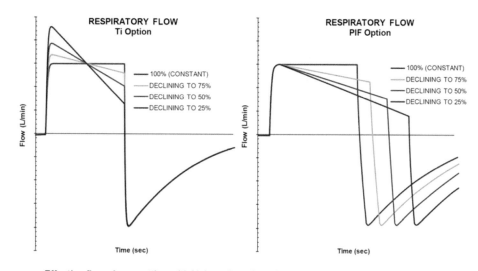

Effective flow shape setting with Volume breath option set to Ti and PIF for a fixed volume

The figure illustrates how Flow Shape affects breath delivery for a fixed volume. With volume breath option set to PIF (Peak Inspiratory Flow), adjusting the flow shape alters the inspiratory duration, whereas with volume breath option set to Ti (Inspiratory time), adjusting the flow shape alters the Peak Inspiratory Flow.

When the flow shape is set to 100%, the flow is generally constant during inspiration. For decreasing percentages, the flow starts at the peak flow and declines to approximately the percentage setting of this value at the end of inspiration.

To select between Ti and PIF options:

1. From the Setup menu select Device config.
2. Select Units
3. Select Ti of PIF.

Monitoring the Patient

Once I have brought the patient in for the initial setup period, I will start adjusting the pressure based on the patient's comfort and also on the monitoring screen. I will depress the 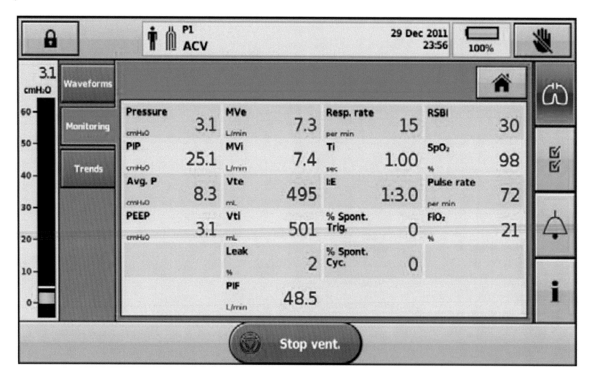 on the right side of the menu and then press the Monitoring on the left-hand side.

Once I have a patient on the machine and being adjusted, I can monitor and adjust for comfort and pressures by going between the monitoring menu and the settings by toggling between these two buttons. I will have the patient lie on a recliner and place the head of the recliner back to allow for a more supine body position. I have also been using the web-based monitoring provided by ResMed. The website Airview.Resmed. com allows one to follow all their patients on the ResMed AirSense platforms and the Astral devices. I have been employing this in my clinical practice and have been allowing patients the freedom to call or to email me issues with their PAP therapy machines, which I will adjust over the website. However, the Astral is considered a ventilator and is not capable of being changed over the internet. Patients will bring me their Astral, or I'll have the DME change their machines after I have downloaded their information.

The Trilogy

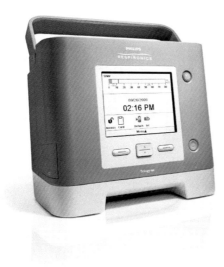

The Trilogy is made by Philips Respironics. The machine has been commonly used in the hospital and in an outpatient setting; however, many physicians don't know how to access this machine. If the machine is on, holding down the alarm button (2) and the down arrow for scrolling (3) will allow one to access the menu. For those who adjust or look at these machines that are off, I suggest turning on the machine and then turning it off quickly and then holding down the alarm button and the down arrow. This way, the machine will not be alarming and will not blow up during the setup process.

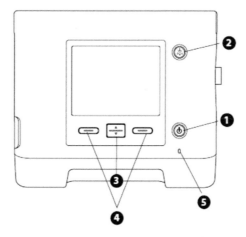

This is the next screen that will appear:

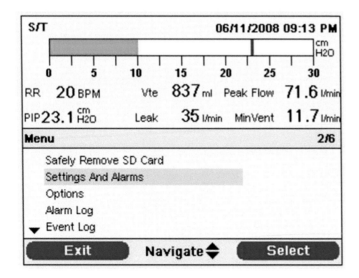 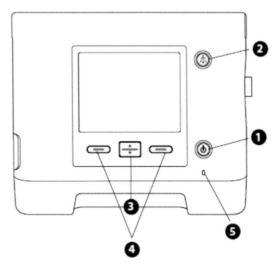

Scroll down with button 3 to the settings, and then select by pressing button 4 to help navigate through the menu. Once you have scrolled down to the Settings and Alarms tab, you can then navigate into this menu by using button 4.

This is the next menu:

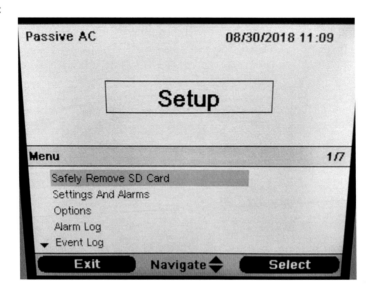

Then scroll down to the Settings and Alarms using the down arrow on button 3. The next screen will be the following diagram. On this screen, scroll down with button 3 to mode, press the right button 4, and enter this selection. Then scroll up or down with button 3 until the mode that is desired is seen, and then select it with the right button 4.

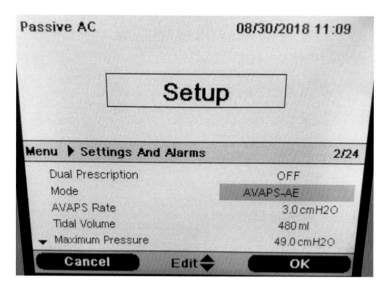

In this menu, the mode is highlighted. Then use button 3 to get to the mode and then button 4 to select. And then press button 3 again to navigate to the different available modes to choose from. Once the AVAPS-AE mode is selected, you can then use buttons 3 and 4 to adjust the parameters for this mode.

AVAPS Rate

The AVAPS rate setting allows you to adjust the maximum rate at which the pressure support automatically changes to achieve the target tidal volume. A higher rate allows the AVAPS algorithm to change pressure support faster to meet the target tidal volume.

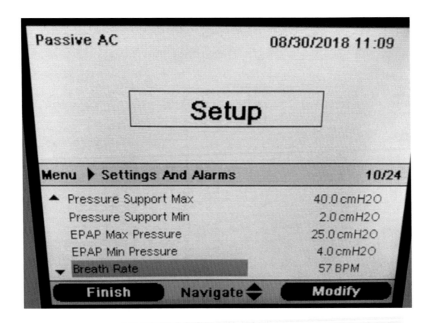

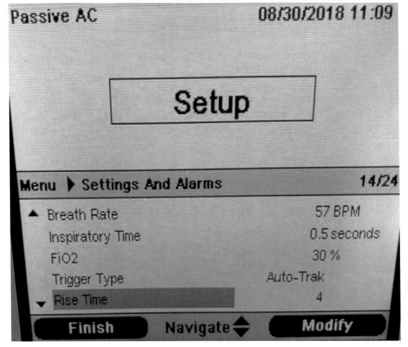

Other Settings

The other setting that needs to be adjusted is the tidal volume; this is the target volume that the machine is being instructed to achieve. The EPAP is adjusted to minimum and maximum values. This can be refined as much as the patient requires in follow-up appointments. The maximum pressure is the pressure that can be achieved by the Trilogy, which includes the EPAP and maximum pressure support supplied by the Trilogy to achieve the given tidal volume. The pressure support is then adjusted with a minimum and maximum allowed pressure to achieve the given tidal volume. Inspiratory time and breath rate also need to be set. The rise time is time during the change from expiratory pressure to inspiratory pressure (levels 1–6).

Other Comfort Features

1. Trigger

   - Flow versus Auto-Trak versus Auto-Trak Sensitivity
     - Flow
       - Set flow trigger at 1–9 L/m.
       - Set flow cycle at 10%–90%.
     - Auto-Trak and Auto-Trak Sensitivity
       - This is computer-generated to respond to patient need.

2. Digital Auto-Trak Sensitivity has the ability to recognize and compensate leaks and automatically adjust its trigger and cycle to maintain performance.

3. Flow trigger sensitivity is the start of inspiration.

4. Flow cycle sensitivity turns on when the flow trigger is on, and this works with expiration.

Monitoring and Compliance of the Patient

Respironics is in the process of upgrading their cloud to help with monitoring the DreamStation and the Trilogy. However, at this time, the Trilogy can be downloaded to paper copy through DirectView.

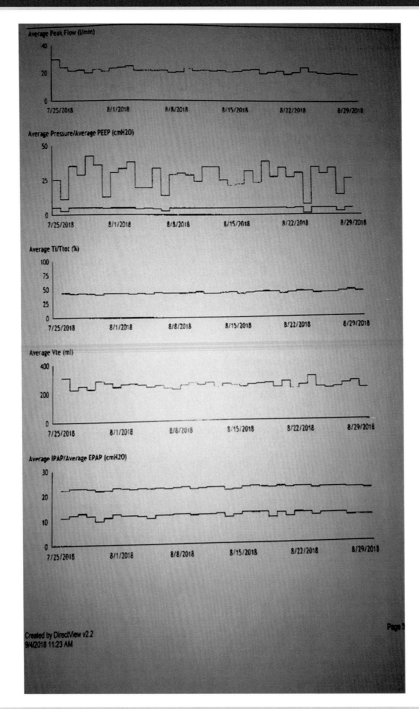

Patterns of Usage

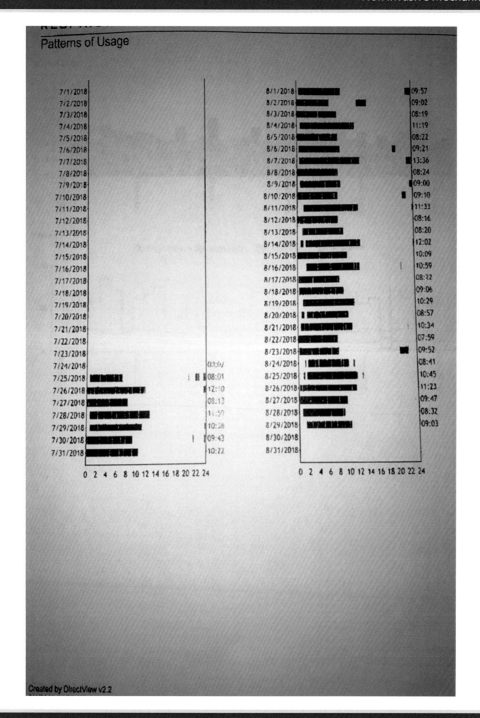

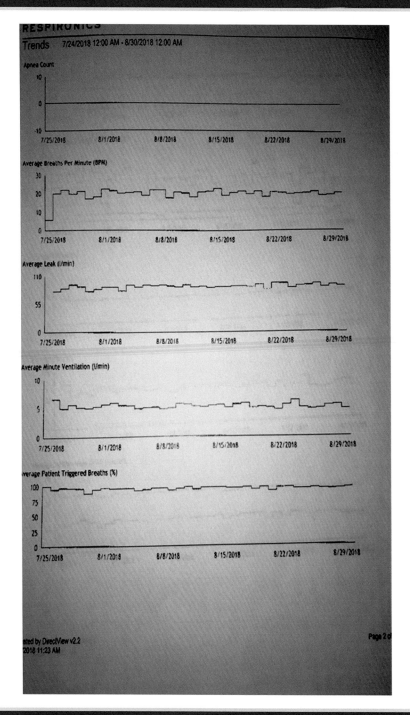

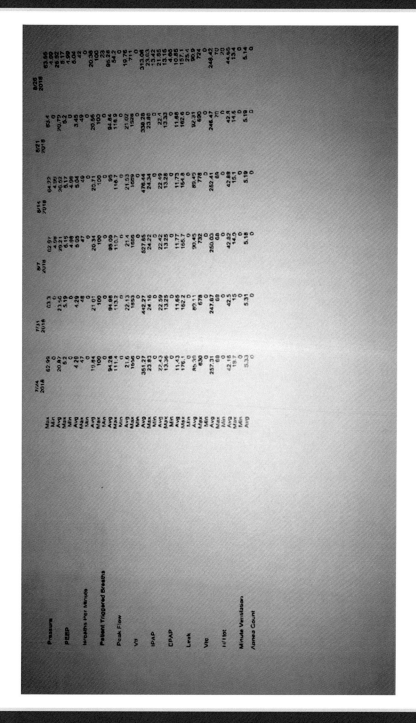

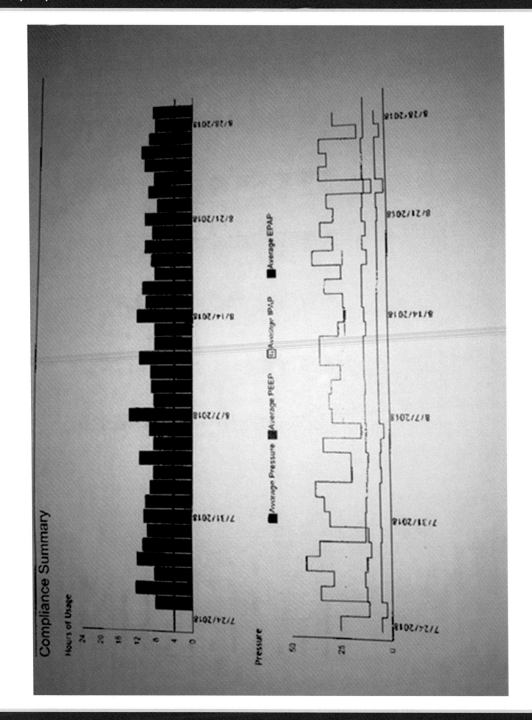

CHAPTER 6
Troubleshooting

1. Patient complains about leaking on the eyes after one hour of use with a full mask. Answer: Change the mask to nasal mask or pillows, which may also need lowering of the pressure.

2. Patient complains about waking up with bloating and/or burping. Answer: Lower the pressure of positive airway pressure or the pressure support or the TVa volumes.

3. ResMed: Patient has issues with lower pressure upon awakening in the middle of the night. Answer: Turn off the auto ramp feature.

4. Patient complains about needing more time to breathe in. Answer: Increase the Ti Max up to 3.0, or slow down the rise time to 400–500 ms.

5. Trilogy: knowing the difference in Trigger/Cycle issues. Auto-Trak vs Auto-Trak Sensitivity.

6. Astral: AHI is > 5. Answer: Increase the EPAP to adjust for this.

7. Astral: AHI is > 5. Answer: Switch iVAPS AE, which is the R6 upgrade.

8. Astral: Leak is high. Answer: Decrease the PS minimum or reduce the TVa volumes.

Resources

1. Garcia Santos de Andrade, Rafaela et al. "Impact of the Type of Mask on the Effectiveness of and Adherence to Continuous Positive Airway Pressure Treatment for Obstructive Sleep Apnea." *J Bras Pneumol* 40, no. 6 (2014): 658–668.

2. NPPV Titration Task Force of the AASM. "Clinical Practices for the Sleep Center Adjustment of Noninvasive Positive Pressure Ventilation (NPPV) in Stable Chronic Alveolar Hypoventilation Syndromes." *Journal of Clinical Sleep Medicine* 5, no. 5 (2010).

3. Despande, Sheetal et al. "Oronasal Masks Require a Higher Pressure than Nasal and Nasal Pillow Mask for the Treatment of Obstructive Sleep Apnea." *Journal of Clinical Sleep Medicine* 12, no. 9 (2016).

4. Bettinzoli, M. et al. "Oronasal Masks Require Higher Levels of Positive Airway Pressure than Nasal Masks to Treat Obstructive Sleep Apnea." *Sleep and Breathing* 18, no. 4 (December 2014): 845–9.

5. Ebben, M. R. et al. "A Randomized Controlled Trial on the Effect of Mask Choice on Residual Respiratory Events with Continuous Positive Airway Pressure Treatment." *Sleep Med* 15, no. 6 (June 2014): 619–24.

6. Salturk, C. et al. "Comparison of Exercise Capacity in COPD and Other Etiologies of Chronic Respiratory Failure Requiring Non-invasive Mechanical Ventilation at Home: Retrospective Analysis of 1-Year Follow-Up." *International Journal of COPD* 10 (November 2015): 2559–2569.

7. Murata, Shinya et al. "Effects of Inspiratory Rise Time on Triggering Work Load during Pressure Support Ventilation: A Lung Model Study." *Respiratory Care* 55, no. 7 (July 2010): 878–884.

8. https://www.resmed.com/us/en/healthcare-professional/products/innovation-and-technology/ventilation-innovation-and-technology.html.

9. ResMed Corp. "Astral Clinical Guide."

10. Chai-Coetzer, C. L. et al. "Continuous Positive Airway Pressure Delivery Interfaces for Obstructive Sleep Apnoea (Review)." *Cochrane Database of Systematic Reviews* no. 4 (2006). Art. no. CD005308.

11. Murphy, P. B. et al. "Effect of Home Noninvasive Ventilation with Oxygen Therapy vs Oxygen Therapy Alone on Hospital Readmission or Death After an Acute COPD Exacerbation." *JAMA* 317, no. 21 (2017): 2177–2186.

12. Philips Respironics Inc. "Trilogy 100 Clinical Manual." REF 10066819, 1072847, JJB (03/10/2011). 1001 Murray Ridge Lane. Murrysville, PA 15668.

13. Chirico, G et al. "Nasal obstruction in neonates and infants." *Minerva Peadiatr.* 2010 Oct;62(5): 499-505

14. Chai-Coetzer CL et al. "Continuous positive airway pressure delivery interfaces for obstructive sleep apnoea (Review)." *Cochrane Database of Systematic Reviews* 2006, Issue 4. Art. No.: CD005308

Printed in the United States
By Bookmasters